About the NCCN Guidelir

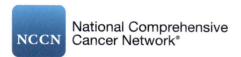
National Comprehensive
Cancer Network®

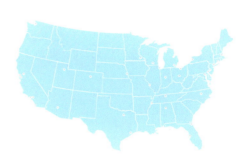

Did you know that top cancer centers across the United States work together to improve cancer care? This alliance of leading cancer centers is called the National Comprehensive Cancer Network® (NCCN®).

Cancer care is always changing. NCCN develops evidence-based cancer care recommendations used by health care providers worldwide. These frequently updated recommendations are the NCCN Clinical Practice Guidelines in Oncology (NCCN Guidelines®). The NCCN Guidelines for Patients plainly explain these expert recommendations for people with cancer and caregivers.

These NCCN Guidelines for Patients are based on the NCCN Clinical Practice Guidelines in Oncology (NCCN Guidelines®) for Rectal Cancer, Version 1.2024 — January 29, 2024.

View the NCCN Guidelines for Patients free online NCCN.org/patientguidelines	Find an NCCN Cancer Center near you NCCN.org/cancercenters

Connect with us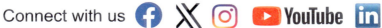

Supporters

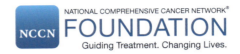

NCCN Guidelines for Patients are supported by funding from the NCCN Foundation®

NCCN Foundation gratefully acknowledges the following corporate supporters for helping to make available these NCCN Guidelines for Patients: Amgen Inc., Exact Sciences, Pfizer Inc., and Taiho Oncology, Inc.

NCCN independently adapts, updates, and hosts the NCCN Guidelines for Patients. Our corporate supporters do not participate in the development of the NCCN Guidelines for Patients and are not responsible for the content and recommendations contained therein.

Additional support is provided by

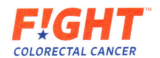

Fight Colorectal Cancer (Fight CRC) is a leading patient-empowerment and advocacy organization providing balanced and objective information on colon and rectal cancer research, treatment, and policy. Serving as relentless champions of hope, focused on funding promising, high-impact research endeavors while equipping advocates to influence legislation and policy for the collective good. Learn more at FightCRC.org, and follow on social media @FightCRC!

To make a gift or learn more, visit online or email

NCCNFoundation.org/donate

PatientGuidelines@NCCN.org

Contents

NCCN Foundation seeks to support the millions of patients and their families affected by a cancer diagnosis by funding and distributing NCCN Guidelines for Patients. NCCN Foundation is also committed to advancing cancer treatment by funding the nation's promising doctors at the center of innovation in cancer research. For more details and the full library of patient and caregiver resources, visit NCCN.org/patients.

National Comprehensive Cancer Network (NCCN) and NCCN Foundation
3025 Chemical Road, Suite 100, Plymouth Meeting, PA 19462 USA

1
Rectal cancer basics

Rectal cancer is common and treatable. Many cancers that start in the rectum can be cured, especially when found and treated early. This guide describes treatment for adenocarcinoma, the most common type of rectal tumor.

The rectum

The rectum is the last several inches of the large intestine (bowel). After digested food becomes stool in the colon, it is held in the rectum until it exits the body through the anus.

The rectal wall is made of layers of tissue. Cancer starts in the innermost layer that comes in contact with stool. If left untreated, cancer cells grow through the layers of the rectal wall, towards the inside of the pelvis. The cancer can then invade structures or organs outside of the rectum. Cancer cells can also break off from the rectal tumor. They can travel through lymph or blood to nearby lymph nodes or to distant organs like the liver or the lungs.

The term colorectal cancer is used to describe cancers that form in either the colon or rectum. While these cancers are similar, their treatment is different. The focus of this guide is rectal cancer. For information on colon cancer treatment, see the *NCCN Guidelines for Patients: Colon Cancer* at NCCN.org/patientguidelines and on the NCCN Patient Guides for Cancer app.

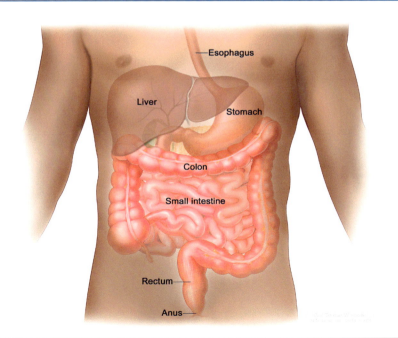

The rectum

The rectum is about 5 inches (12 centimeters) long and forms the last part of the large bowel. Stool is held in the rectum until it leaves the body through the anus.

Polyps

Polyps are non-cancerous growths that form on the inner lining of the colon and rectum. The most common type is called an adenoma. While it may take many years, adenomas can become invasive rectal cancer. Cancer that forms in an adenoma is called an adenocarcinoma. This is the most common type of rectal cancer. Polyps that rarely turn into cancer include hyperplastic and inflammatory polyps.

While most polyps do not become cancer, almost all rectal cancers start in a polyp. Removing polyps can prevent cancer before it starts. Most can be removed during a colonoscopy using a minor surgical procedure called a polypectomy. Polyps can also be tested to make sure that cancer hasn't already started to form.

For more information on finding polyps early, see the *NCCN Guidelines for Patients: Colorectal Cancer Screening* at NCCN.org/ patientguidelines and on the NCCN Patient Guides for Cancer app.

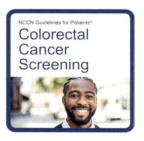

Key points

> The rectum is the last part of the large bowel. Stool is held in the rectum until it leaves the body through the anus.

> Polyps are non-cancerous growths that form on the inner lining of the colon and rectum.

> Most rectal cancers start in polyps called adenomas. These cancers are called adenocarcinomas.

2
Testing and treatment planning

This chapter discusses testing and other steps needed to create your treatment plan.

Mismatch repair testing

Everyone diagnosed with rectal cancer should have their tumor tested for mutations (changes) in genes that fix damaged DNA, called mismatch repair (MMR) genes. This feature of some rectal cancers is a type of biomarker. Biomarkers are targetable changes of a cancer that can help guide treatment.

Testing involves analyzing a piece of the rectal tumor in a lab. Depending on the method used, an abnormal result is called either:

> ➤ mismatch repair deficient (dMMR) or microsatellite instability-high (MSI-H).

Tumors that do not have these changes are referred to as:

> ➤ microsatellite stable (MSS) or mismatch repair proficient (pMMR).

If the cancer is dMMR/MSI-H, you will also be tested for inherited mutations in the mismatch repair genes (explained next).

Family health history

Most rectal cancers occur for unknown reasons. While rare, some people are born with a gene mutation that makes them more likely to get rectal and other cancers. People born with Lynch syndrome, for example, are at high risk of developing colorectal, endometrial, and ovarian cancers.

Lynch syndrome is caused by inherited mutations in the mismatch repair (MMR) genes. Everyone diagnosed with rectal cancer should have their tumor tested for mutations in the MMR genes. If the cancer is dMMR/MSI-H, you will also be tested for Lynch syndrome.

Familial adenomatous polyposis (FAP) is another rare inherited cancer syndrome. FAP can cause hundreds to thousands of polyps to form in the colon and rectum. The polyps start as benign growths, but over time can become invasive rectal cancer.

There are other inherited syndromes that are even more rare than Lynch syndrome and FAP.

If your provider thinks you may have an inherited syndrome, they will refer you to a genetic counselor. This expert can talk with you and your family about getting tested for syndromes related to rectal cancer. If they determine that testing is appropriate, they can order a blood or saliva test to see if you have an inherited gene mutation.

Blood tests

General health tests

A complete blood count (CBC) measures the number of white blood cells, red blood cells, and platelets in a blood sample. White blood cells help you fight infection. Red blood cells carry oxygen throughout the body. Platelets help wounds heal by forming blood clots.

A chemistry profile (also called a comprehensive metabolic panel), is a group of tests that provides information about how well your kidneys, liver, and other organs are working.

CEA blood test

Carcinoembryonic antigen (CEA) is a protein found in blood. People with colorectal cancer tend to have more than normal. Monitoring CEA can be helpful for some cancers that are only in the rectum. If the level rises, it could signal that the cancer has spread. If the level is high at diagnosis, it could suggest that the cancer has already spread. Monitoring CEA isn't helpful for everyone. Pregnant people and tobacco users may also have more CEA than average in their blood.

Write everything down and keep a binder or folder of information. If your loved one wakes up violently ill at midnight, it's after hours and you need to know who to call. Be prepared before that happens, so you don't have to scramble in an emergency. Have all phone numbers in one place (even if it's on your phone)."

ctDNA

There is growing interest in circulating tumor DNA (ctDNA) testing for colorectal cancer. Also called a liquid biopsy, this test looks for small pieces of DNA released by tumor cells into the blood. It can detect microscopic rectal cancer cells that may remain in the body after treatment. This may become helpful for predicting whether the cancer is likely to return. **But, at this time, ctDNA testing is still being studied in clinical trials.**

Imaging

Imaging tests can show areas of cancer inside the body. This information helps your care team stage the cancer and plan treatment. A radiologist will interpret and convey the imaging results to your oncologist.

Your care team will tell you how to prepare for these tests. You may need to stop taking some medicines and stop eating and drinking for a few hours beforehand.

Some imaging tests use contrast. Contrast is a substance that makes the pictures clearer. It is injected into your vein and/or mixed with a liquid to drink. Tell your doctor if you've had problems with contrast in the past. You may be given or advised to take a steroid and an antihistamine medication (like Benadryl) before the scan. It will lower the risk of an allergic reaction.

MRI

If surgery is needed or being considered, your doctor will order magnetic resonance imaging (MRI) of your pelvis. MRI can show how deep into the rectal wall the cancer has grown and whether it has spread to nearby lymph nodes. Special techniques called a staging protocol are used to stage the cancer. Contrast may or may not be used.

MRI doesn't use radiation and is safe for most people. People with certain heart monitors, pacemakers, or some types of surgical clips generally can't have MRI. Tell your team if you get nervous in small spaces. You may be given a sedative (medicine) to help you relax.

In some cases, MRI may be used to look for cancer in the abdomen, especially the liver. This may be the case if you can't have the contrast agent used for a CT scan.

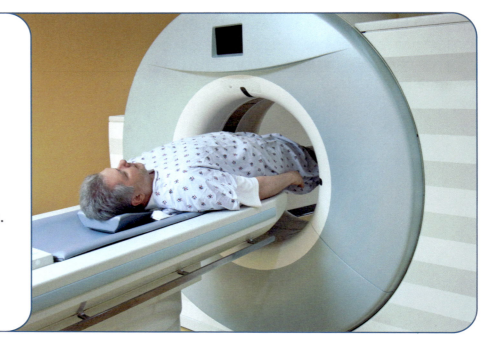

MRI

An MRI can show how deep into the rectal wall the cancer has grown and whether it has spread to nearby lymph nodes.

A gel may be inserted into the rectum before MRI imaging. A light coil device or blanket will be placed on top of you. It sends and receives radio waves to record the images. The device covers your body from below your chest to the top of your legs. Straps may be used to help you stay in place. You may feel a bit warm during the scan.

Endorectal ultrasound

While a pelvic MRI is preferred for imaging rectal cancer, an endorectal ultrasound (EUS) is sometimes performed instead. Using sound waves, this test can also show the extent of cancer in the pelvis. A small probe is inserted into the rectum. Echoes form a picture that can be seen by your doctor on a screen. If needed, EUS may also be used to guide a biopsy of lymph nodes or other areas near the rectum.

CT

A computed tomography (CT) scan of your chest and abdomen is recommended as part of initial testing. CT can show if the cancer has spread to the liver, lungs, or other organs. Contrast will be used. During the scan you will lie face-up on a table that moves through a tunnel-like machine. A technician will be nearby. You will be able to hear and talk to them at all times.

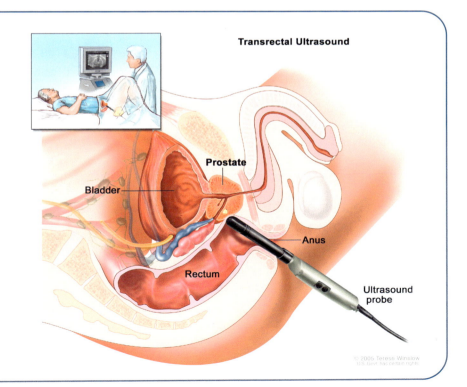

Transrectal Ultrasound

Endorectal ultrasound

If you can't have a pelvic MRI (because you have a pacemaker, for example) or if MRI images were unhelpful, you may have an endorectal ultrasound instead. This test may also be ordered if your doctor knows the cancer has not grown far into the rectal wall.

Prostate

Bladder

Anus

Rectum

Ultrasound probe

© 2005 Terese Winslow
U.S. Govt. has certain rights

Fertility and family planning

For unknown reasons, colorectal cancer is being diagnosed more often in young adults. Some cancer treatments make it hard or impossible to have children. Radiation therapy, for example, is used to treat many rectal cancers. Radiation damages the hormone-making function of the ovaries and testicles. This can cause the inability to conceive a child.

Damage to the ovaries is known as premature ovarian insufficiency (POI) or radiation-induced premature menopause. See the *Survivorship* chapter of this guide for more information on this side effect.

If you want the option of having children after treatment or are unsure, tell your care team. Your doctor will discuss any fertility-related risks of your treatment plan with you. You may be referred for counseling about your fertility preservation options. Some are described next.

Sperm banking

Sperm banking stores semen for later use by freezing it in liquid nitrogen. The medical term for this is semen cryopreservation.

Egg freezing

Like sperm banking, unfertilized eggs can be removed, frozen, and stored for later use. The medical term for this is oocyte cryopreservation.

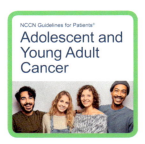

For more information on fertility and family planning, see the *NCCN Guidelines for Patients for Adolescent and Young Adult Cancer* at NCCN.org/ patientguidelines and on the NCCN Patient Guides for Cancer app.

Ovarian tissue banking

This method involves removing part or all of an ovary and freezing the part that contains the eggs. The frozen tissue that contains the eggs can later be unfrozen and put back in the body.

Ovarian transposition

Rectal cancer treatment may involve external beam radiation therapy (EBRT). Radiation damages the ovaries and causes them to stop producing hormones needed for natural pregnancy. Ovarian transposition is a surgery that moves one or both ovaries out of the range of the radiation beam. The medical name for this procedure is oophoropexy.

Key points

- All rectal tumors should be tested for mismatch repair deficiency (dMMR) or high microsatellite instability (MSI-H).

- For cancers with this biomarker, testing for an inherited cancer syndrome called Lynch syndrome is recommended.

- Cancers that don't have this biomarker are called mismatch repair proficient (pMMR) or microsatellite stable (MSS).

- Everyone with rectal cancer should be asked about their family health history.

- MRI of the pelvis using a rectal cancer staging technique can show the extent of the cancer in the rectum and nearby lymph nodes.

- CT of the chest and abdomen can show if the cancer has spread to the liver, lungs, or other organs.

- If you want the option of having children in the future, or are unsure, tell your care team. Your doctor will inform you of any fertility-related risks of your treatment plan and your options for preserving fertility.

When you're up at 1 am, don't "Dr. Google." Go to reputable sites that have patient/caregiver information and resources. Recent, medically reviewed resources are more valuable than random Google results."

3

Treatment for non-metastatic cancer

Rectal cancer often forms in polyps on the lining of the rectum, but can also form as lesions. This chapter explains treatment for rectal cancer that hasn't spread to areas far from the rectum.

Polyps with cancer

A polyp is an overgrowth of cells on the inner lining of the rectal wall. Adenomas are the most common type. While it may take many years, they can become invasive cancer. Cancer that forms in an adenoma is called an adenocarcinoma.

There are 2 main shapes of polyps. Pedunculated polyps are shaped like mushrooms and stick out from the colon wall. They have a stalk and round top. Sessile polyps are flatter and do not have a stalk. A polyp in which cancer has just started to grow is called a malignant (cancerous) polyp.

Most polyps can be removed during a colonoscopy, using a minor surgical procedure called a polypectomy. Often, no further

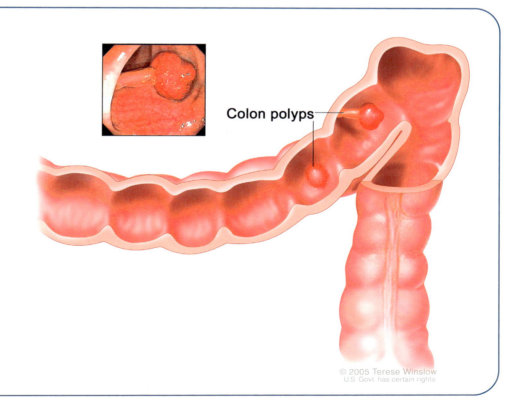

Polyps

Polyps are growths on the lining of the bowel wall. Pedunculated polyps look like mushrooms and stick out from the colon wall. Sessile polyps are flatter and don't have a stalk.

Colon polyps

© 2005 Terese Winslow
U.S. Govt. has certain rights

treatment is needed. In other cases, resection (surgical removal) of a larger piece of the rectum is needed. This depends on the following factors:

> The size and shape of the polyp

> The polypectomy results

> The results of testing the removed tissue

Before deciding whether resection is needed after a polypectomy, your provider will review the results of testing with you and discuss your options. Sessile polyps are more likely to return after treatment. Imaging with endoscopic ultrasound (EUS) or pelvic magnetic resonance imaging (MRI) is recommended for these polyps to help guide decisions about surgery.

Early rectal cancer

If cancer that formed in a polyp isn't found early enough to be removed by polypectomy, surgery is needed. Surgery is also needed for rectal cancer that forms as a lesion on the rectal wall.

The true extent of the cancer can't be known until after surgery. But it can be estimated based on certain test results. This best guess is called the clinical or pre-surgery stage. It is used to determine your treatment options.

Endoscopic submucosal dissection

If testing finds that the tumor hasn't grown beyond the second (muscle) layer of the rectal wall, it is a **T1** tumor. Endoscopic submucosal dissection (ESD) is a recommended option for all T1 tumors. This minimally invasive procedure removes small rectal cancers in one piece, often curing them. Another name for this procedure is endoscopic mucosal resection (EMR).

First, an endoscope is used to locate the tumor in the rectal wall. A tool is guided through the scope to inject fluid between the tumor and the layer of muscle beneath it. This helps lift and separate the tumor, making it easier to cut off. Most people don't need more treatment.

Surveillance after ESD
Checking for recurrence is recommended for at least 5 years after ESD. During this time you will have flexible sigmoidoscopy about every 6 months. The first one may be as early as 3 months after ESD.

Imaging with endorectal ultrasound or pelvic MRI (with contrast) is recommended every 3 to 6 months for the first 2 years, then every 6 months through the fifth year.

Transanal local excision

For **T1** tumors located at the end of the rectum, removing them through the anus may be an option. This is called transanal local excision.

The surgeon cuts through all layers of the rectal wall to remove the cancer and some surrounding normal rectal tissue. Lymph nodes are not removed.

Advanced techniques for removing tumors higher in the rectum include transanal endoscopic microsurgery (TEM) and transanal minimally invasive surgery (TAMIS).

If surgery confirms that the cancer is T1 and the tumor is considered low risk, no further treatment is needed. Surveillance will begin.

Surveillance after transanal local excision

Proctoscopies and imaging are recommended for 5 years after transanal local excision. These will take place every 3 to 6 months for the first 2 years, then every 6 months the next 3 years. For the imaging, either endorectal ultrasound or MRI with contrast is recommended.

A colonoscopy is recommended 1 year after surgery. If the results are good, your next colonoscopy will take place in 3 years. After that, a colonoscopy is recommended every 5 years.

Other local excision results

Sometimes more treatment is needed after local excision. Reasons you may need more treatment include:

> Testing of the removed tissues finds high-risk features

> The tumor is larger than expected and has invaded the muscle layer (a T2 tumor)

In either case, the **preferred** next treatment is transabdominal surgery. See the next page for more information on this method.

A second option is chemotherapy combined with radiation. Doctors call this chemoradiation. This treatment approach is normally used for locally advanced cancers. See page 23 for more information. If chemoradiation works well, you might have chemotherapy next to kill any lingering cancer cells. Or, you and your doctor may agree to watch and wait.

If there are signs of cancer after chemoradiation, transabdominal resection is recommended. Chemotherapy may follow.

Transabdominal surgery

Transabdominal surgery is recommended for tumors that have invaded the muscle layer of the rectal wall. In staging terms, these are T2 tumors. Abdominal surgery is also a recommended option for:

> smaller (T1) tumors, and

> some larger (T3) cancers that haven't spread to lymph nodes.

This method involves cutting into the abdomen to reach and remove the rectal tumor, some surrounding healthy tissue, and nearby lymph nodes. A pathologist examines the removed tissue and determines the cancer stage.

The type of transabdominal surgery performed depends on the location of the tumor and the extent of the cancer. At least 12 lymph nodes should be removed during all types of transabdominal surgery.

Low anterior resection

A low anterior resection (LAR) is a type of transabdominal surgery used for tumors in the mid to upper rectum.

In addition to the rectal tumor, part or all of the last section of the colon is removed. When possible, the colon is connected to the remaining rectum. This is called a colorectal anastomosis (reconnection). Otherwise the colon may be attached directly to the anus. This is called a coloanal anastomosis. This

---

Low anterior resection (LAR)

LAR is a type of abdominal surgery used to remove tumors in the mid to upper rectum. The rectal tumor and part or all of the sigmoid colon is removed. When possible, the colon is connected to the remaining rectum.

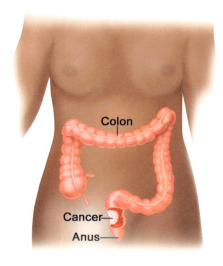
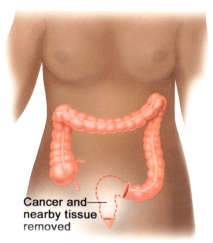
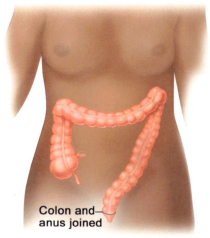

allows for the possibility of having near-normal bowel movements.

Your surgeon is likely to delay reattaching the bowel in order to let the surgical site heal. In this case, or if the colon can't be connected to the anus, a colostomy is made. A colostomy connects a part of the colon to the outside of the abdomen. This creates an opening (a stoma) on the surface of the abdomen. Stool exits the body through the stoma and goes into a bag attached to the skin. A colostomy may only be needed for a short time to allow the rectum to heal before being reconnected to the colon. But sometimes it is needed permanently.

Abdominoperineal resection

This type of transabdominal surgery is used for tumors in the lower rectum. These tumors may have grown into the anus or nearby pelvic floor muscle (levator ani).

Abdominoperineal resection (APR) typically involves removing the anus, the rectum, the area where the rectum and colon meet, and other tissue. In some cases, the levator muscles are also removed. The outer ring of muscle in the anus may be spared. A permanent colostomy is always needed.

Abdominoperineal resection (APR)

APR is used for tumors in the lower rectum that may have grown into the anus or nearby muscle. It involves removing the rectum and anus and creating a permanent colostomy for stool to leave the body.

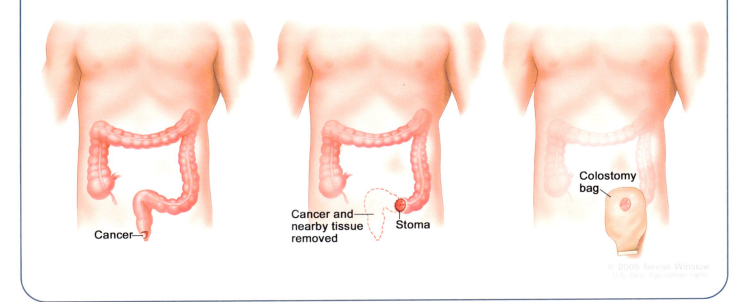

Cancer

Cancer and nearby tissue removed   Stoma

Colostomy bag

After transabdominal surgery

The tissue and lymph nodes removed during surgery are sent to a lab for testing.

A pathologist assesses how far the cancer has grown within the rectal wall and whether any removed lymph nodes have cancer. Using this information, they assign the cancer a stage of I (1), II (2), or III (3). This process is called surgical (or pathologic) staging. The stage is used to determine whether more treatment is needed.

In stage 1, the tumor has grown into the second or third (muscle) layer of the rectal wall. No further treatment is needed.

In stage 2, the tumor has grown through the rectal wall and possibly into nearby tissues or organs. In stage 3, cancer has spread to nearby lymph nodes. More treatment is almost always needed for stage 2 and 3 cancers. Next treatments may include chemoradiation,

chemotherapy, or both. More information on chemotherapy is provided next. See page 24 for information on chemoradiation.

Chemotherapy

Chemotherapy is given in cycles of treatment days followed by days of rest. This allows your body to recover between cycles. Cycles vary in length depending on which drugs are used. Chemotherapy regimens used to treat rectal cancer are listed in **Guide 1**.

Any regimen that has "OX" in the name includes oxaliplatin. Oxaliplatin can cause nerve damage (called neuropathy) to your fingers and toes. Symptoms include numbness, cramping, tingling, or pain in these areas.

Any regimen that has "IRI" in the name contains irinotecan. Irinotecan tends to cause abdominal cramping, nausea, diarrhea, and hair loss.

Guide 1 Chemotherapy regimens	
FOLFOX	Folinic acid (leucovorin calcium) + fluorouracil + oxaliplatin
CAPEOX	Capecitabine + oxaliplatin
FOLFIRI	Folinic acid (leucovorin calcium) + fluorouracil + irinotecan
FOLFIRINOX	Folinic acid (leucovorin calcium) + fluorouracil + irinotecan + oxaliplatin
5-FU/LV	Fluorouracil + folinic acid (leucovorin calcium)
Capecitabine	Capecitabine

If regimens containing oxaliplatin and/or irinotecan are expected to be too harsh, your doctor may recommend 5-FU/leucovorin or capecitabine. These regimens also have side effects. Capecitabine can cause hand-foot syndrome. Symptoms include redness, swelling, and pain on the palms of the hands, bottoms of the feet, or both. Sometimes blisters appear.

Surveillance after transabdominal surgery

For cancers found to be **stage 1** by surgical staging, colonoscopy is recommended in 1 year. If the results are good, the next will take place in 3 years. After that, colonoscopy is recommended every 5 years until you and your doctor agree to stop.

If you don't have any symptoms, other testing isn't needed on a regular basis. Your provider may order imaging tests if they suspect the cancer has returned or spread.

For cancers found to be **stage 2 or 3** by surgical staging, surveillance includes physical exams, colonoscopies, carcinoembryonic antigen (CEA) blood tests, and computed tomography (CT) scans. The recommended schedule for this testing is shown in **Guide 2**.

In addition to surveillance testing, a range of other care is important for cancer survivors. See the *Survivorship* chapter of this patient guide for more information.

Guide 2 Surveillance after transabdominal surgery – stage 2 and 3 cancers	
Physical exam and CEA blood test	**First 2 years:** Every 3 to 6 months **Next 3 years:** Every 6 months
CT of chest, abdomen, and pelvis	Every 6 to 12 months for 5 years
Colonoscopy	**You did not have a total colonoscopy at diagnosis:** Colonoscopy is recommended 3 to 6 months after surgery. **You had a total colonoscopy at diagnosis:** Colonoscopy is recommended 1 year after surgery. If no advanced adenomas are found, repeat in 3 years. After that, repeat every 5 years.

Locally advanced cancer

The term locally advanced is used to describe rectal cancers that:

> have grown through the rectal wall (a T3 or T4 tumor), or

> have spread to nearby lymph nodes, or

> can't be removed using surgery.

Treatment depends on the mismatch repair (MMR) status of the cancer and often involves external beam radiation therapy (EBRT) and chemoradiation.

In EBRT, radiation is delivered using a large machine outside the body. The radiation passes through skin and other tissue to reach the tumor. The radiation beams are shaped to the cancer site. This helps minimize damage to healthy tissue. There are different types of EBRT. The type used depends on the location and size of the tumor(s) and other factors.

Long-course chemoradiation

EBRT is often used with chemotherapy to treat rectal cancer. This is known as long-course chemoradiation. Radiation therapy is given in 25 to 28 treatment sessions, called fractions. Most people have 5 sessions per week.

Chemotherapy is given during the same period. When given with radiation, chemotherapy can make it easier for radiation to kill cancer cells. This is called radiosensitizing chemotherapy.

Long-course chemoradiation

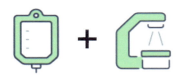

- 25 to 28 radiation treatment sessions (Monday through Friday)
- Chemotherapy is given during the same time period
- Either 5-fluorouracil or capecitabine is usually given for chemotherapy

Short-course radiation therapy

- High-dose radiation is given over a short time period
- Typically only 5 treatment sessions are needed

For many years, long-course chemoradiation was the standard approach for treating locally advanced rectal cancer. Short-course radiation therapy is another option found to have similar outcomes in certain cases.

Either 5-fluorouracil or capecitabine is usually given for chemotherapy. 5-FU is given using an infusion pump hooked into a central access device like a portacath. You take this pump home with you for up to a week at a time. Capecitabine is a pill that you take twice daily on every radiation day.

Short-course radiation therapy

Another method of radiation treatment for rectal cancer is short-course radiation therapy. This method delivers a higher dose of radiation over a much shorter time period, typically in 5 treatment sessions. Chemotherapy is not given.

If external radiation is planned

A planning session (called a CT simulation) is needed before treatment begins. While in the treatment position, a CT scan is performed to take pictures of the cancer site. Devices may be used to keep you from moving, with you sometimes lying on your back or on your stomach. Your radiation team uses these pictures to plan the details of your treatment.

During real sessions, you will lie on a table as you did for simulation. Ink marks are used to precisely position your body in the treatment room. This helps to target the tumor.

A technician will operate the machine from a nearby room. You will be able to hear and speak with them at all times. As treatment is given, you will not see, hear, or feel the radiation. One session can take less than 10 minutes. Sessions may take longer if imaging to verify the position is done before each treatment. This is called image-guided radiation therapy (IGRT).

Side effects of radiation therapy

- Feeling tired and worn out

- Hair loss in the treated area

- Changes to urination and bowel movements

- Diarrhea

- Nausea or vomiting

- Late side effects can include infertility, sexual problems, bowel problems, reduced bone density, and second cancers

- Vaginal dilators can help with sexual problems—see the Survivorship chapter of this guide for more information

- Not all side effects are listed here. Ask your treatment team for a full list.

In this case, the imaging is used to confirm the position of the tumor and the accuracy of the setup. It isn't used to check how well the cancer is responding to treatment.

Treatment for pMMR/MSS cancers

Most locally advanced cancers are treated first with 12 to 16 weeks of chemotherapy **and** either long-course chemoradiation or short-course radiation therapy. In most cases, transabdominal surgery follows. This approach is known as total neoadjuvant therapy (TNT). The order in which you receive these treatments can vary. Your care team will determine the best sequence for you.

After treatment, you will have imaging tests to check the extent of the cancer. This is called restaging. For most people, transabdominal surgery is the recommended next step.

Sometimes, these first treatments work so well that no cancer can be detected in the body. Doctors call this a complete response. If this happens, some research suggests that surgery doesn't always lead to better treatment outcomes. You may be given the option to monitor the cancer closely instead. This is only an option for carefully selected patients who agree to close surveillance programs. **See Guide 3.**

The benefits and risks of taking a watch-and-wait approach instead of having surgery aren't fully known. The decision to have surgery (or not) should be one that you make with your doctor after careful consideration.

Guide 3
Surveillance after non-surgical treatment

Physical exam and CEA blood test	**First 2 years:** Every 3 to 6 months **Next 3 years:** Every 6 months
Digital rectal exam (DRE) and proctoscopy or flexible sigmoidoscopy	**First 2 years:** Every 3 to 4 months **Next 3 years:** Every 6 months
Imaging	MRI of rectum recommended every 6 months for up to 3 years. CT of chest and abdomen recommended every 6 to 12 months for a total of 5 years. When pelvic MRIs stop after 3 years, CT will also include the pelvis.
Colonoscopy	Recommended 1 year after treatment. If no advanced adenomas are found, your next will be in 3 years. After that, colonoscopy is recommended every 5 years.

Treatment for dMMR/MSI-H cancers

There are 2 treatment approaches for cancers with these biomarkers. Immunotherapy, described first below, is preferred.

Immunotherapy

The preferred treatment approach for locally advanced cancers with these biomarkers begins with immunotherapy. At this time, recommended immune checkpoint inhibitors include:

> Nivolumab (Opdivo), which may be given with ipilimumab (Yervoy)

> Pembrolizumab (Keytruda)

> Dostarlimab-gxly (Jemperli)

Immunotherapy is recommended for up to 6 months. The extent of the cancer will be checked every 2 to 3 months during this time. In some cases, no more treatment is needed.

If cancer remains after 6 months of immunotherapy, treatment with long-course chemoradiation or short-course radiation therapy is recommended. Transabdominal resection (surgery) is often the next step. Chemotherapy may follow surgery.

Total neoadjuvant therapy

If you cannot have immunotherapy, a second approach for cancers with these biomarkers is total neoadjuvant therapy.

Treatment begins with either long-course chemoradiation or short-course radiation therapy. The next step is 12 to 16 weeks of chemotherapy. Either FOLFOX or CAPEOX is usually given. After treatment, imaging tests will be ordered to see if transabdominal resection is an option. If cancer remains, surgery is recommended.

Immunotherapy side effects

Immune checkpoint inhibitors have unique side effects. Unlike other cancer treatments, the side effects of immunotherapy occur because the immune system is attacking healthy cells in the body. Learning to recognize possible side effects can help you notice reactions early and report them to your care team.

More information on the side effects of immune checkpoint inhibitors is available at NCCN.org/patientguidelines and on the NCCN Patient Guides for Cancer app.

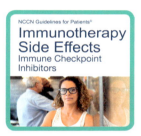

Recurrence

Cancer that returns to the rectum or to nearby areas in the pelvis is called a local recurrence. Treatment options depend on whether the cancer is (or may become) surgically resectable and whether you have had previous radiation to your pelvis.

If the cancer is small enough, your first treatment may be surgery. After surgery, chemoradiation is often given to kill any remaining cancer cells in the pelvis.

In other cases, chemotherapy and either long-course chemoradiation or short-course radiation therapy is given first. The goal is to shrink the cancer enough that it can be removed surgically.

If surgery is not possible, you may have treatment with systemic therapy, chemoradiation, or short-course radiation. If systemic therapy is planned, your doctor will consider the following in order to select an appropriate regimen for you:

> Chemotherapy medicines you've already received

> Whether the tumor has any biomarkers

> How well you are expected to tolerate certain systemic therapies

When cancer returns to areas far from the rectum, it is called a distant recurrence. See the next chapter for information.

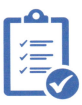

We want your feedback!

Our goal is to provide helpful and easy-to-understand information on cancer.

Take our survey to let us know what we got right and what we could do better.

NCCN.org/patients/feedback

Key points

- After being removed by polypectomy, many polyps don't need more treatment. In other cases, surgery to remove a larger piece of the rectum is needed. Your doctor will review the results of testing with you and discuss your options.

- Surgery is recommended for early rectal cancers when possible. The method used depends on the location and extent of the tumor.

- Treatment options may include endoscopic submucosal dissection (ESD), transanal local excision, and transabdominal surgery. Types of transabdominal surgery include low anterior resection (LAR) and abdominoperineal resection (APR).

- Locally advanced cancers have grown through the rectal wall or have spread to nearby lymph nodes.

- Treatment for locally advanced pMMR cancers starts with chemotherapy and either long-course chemoradiation or short course radiation therapy. Surgery usually follows.

- Immunotherapy is preferred for locally advanced dMMR cancers. Chemoradiation, radiation therapy, and/or surgery may follow. A second option for these cancers involves either chemoradiation or radiation therapy first, followed by chemotherapy alone. Surgery will follow if needed and possible.

4
Treatment for metastatic cancer

Rectal cancer spreads most often to the liver and less often to the lungs, abdomen, or other areas. Treatment for metastatic cancer depends on whether the cancer has the mismatch repair deficiency (dMMR) biomarker.

Biomarker testing

Biomarkers are targetable features of a cancer. Many biomarkers are non-inherited mutations (changes) in the tumor's genes. When possible, biomarker testing is performed on a piece of tumor tissue removed during a biopsy or surgery. If this isn't an option, a sample of blood can be tested instead.

Testing for many biomarkers at one time is called next-generation sequencing (NGS). This preferred method can find rare biomarkers for which targeted treatments may be available. Ideally, all rectal cancers should be tested using NGS to look for the following biomarkers:

> *RAS* (*KRAS* and *NRAS*) mutations

> *BRAF* mutations

> HER2 amplification

> dMMR/MSI-H (if not already performed)

> *POLE/POLD1* mutations

> *RET* fusions

> *NTRK* fusions

Local therapies

Treatment options for rectal cancer may include local therapies. These are treatments that target metastatic liver and lung tumors directly. Some are interventional oncology/radiology techniques, also known as image-guided therapies. These techniques use imaging, such as ultrasound or computed tomography (CT), to deliver minimally invasive cancer treatments. Using imaging during the procedure allows your doctor to precisely target the tumor(s).

A team of experts can determine the best local therapy for your metastatic tumor(s). To learn if surgery or treatment with other local therapies is an option, your case should be evaluated by a multidisciplinary team of experts. The team should include a surgeon experienced in removing liver and lung tumors and an interventional oncologist/radiologist.

Resection

Surgery to remove liver and/or lung tumors is called resection. Resection is often preferred for removing rectal cancer that has spread to these organs.

Image-guided thermal ablation (described next) may be used:

> With resection, if surgery is not expected to completely remove the tumors

> Instead of resection, if the tumors are small and can be completely destroyed

If a liver resection is needed, your liver may need to be enlarged first. This is done using a minimally invasive procedure called portal vein embolization. An interventional radiologist inserts a catheter into certain veins in the liver. This blocks the blood vessel to the liver tumor, causing the healthy part of the liver to grow.

Ablation

Image-guided thermal ablation destroys small liver or lung tumors. A specialized needle is placed directly into or next to the target tumor. This probe delivers targeted energy to the tumor while minimizing damage to surrounding normal tissue.

Radiofrequency and microwave ablation are commonly used methods that kill cancer cells using heat. Cold energy (cryoablation) is used sometimes, mostly for lung tumors. Less common types include irreversible electroporation ("nanoknife") and laser ablation.

Thermal ablation may be used in addition to surgery, or alone for small tumors that can be fully destroyed. It will only be used if all visible areas of cancer can be destroyed. Ablation may be performed by either an interventional radiologist or a surgeon. Sometimes it can be done in a single session in the interventional radiology department.

Liver-directed therapies

Embolization
If the cancer has spread only (or mainly) to the liver, treatment with intra-arterial liver-directed therapies may be an option. These therapies may be considered for liver tumors that:

> Didn't improve (or stopped improving) with chemotherapy, and

> Cannot be resected or ablated.

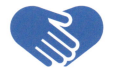

Supportive care is available for everyone with cancer. It isn't meant to treat the cancer, but rather to help with symptoms and make you more comfortable.

Intra-arterial therapies treat liver tumors with chemotherapy beads (chemoembolization) or radioactive spheres (radioembolization). If radiation spheres are used, it is known as selective internal radiation therapy (SIRT) or transarterial hepatic radioembolization (TARE). These procedures are performed by interventional oncologists/radiologists.

A catheter is inserted into an artery in your leg or wrist and guided to the liver tumor(s). Once in place, the spheres or beads are injected into the blood vessel leading to the tumor. They collect inside the tumor and deliver radiation or chemotherapy, causing the cancer cells to die.

The chemotherapy beads can also work to starve the tumor by stopping its blood supply. The chemotherapy beads are larger than the radiation spheres, which means that they block the liver artery in which they are placed. This starves the metastatic tumor by stopping its blood supply. The chemotherapy or radiation further damage the cancer cells and cause the tumor to shrink.

If it isn't safe to use chemotherapy beads, beads that don't contain chemotherapy may be used to physically block blood supply to the tumor. This is called bland embolization.

HAIC

Hepatic arterial infusion chemotherapy (HAIC) is chemotherapy given directly to the liver. It is often given in addition to standard intravenous chemotherapy. Using a port or pump that is usually placed during surgery to remove liver tumors, the drugs are funneled directly into the artery leading to the liver. HAIC should only be performed by medical oncologists at treatment centers with experience in this method.

Stereotactic body radiation therapy

Stereotactic body radiation therapy (SBRT) is a highly specialized type of external radiation therapy. It may be used to treat rectal cancer that has spread to the liver, lungs, or bone.

In SBRT, high doses of radiation are delivered to metastatic tumor(s) using very precise beams. The radiation comes from a large machine outside the body. The radiation passes through skin and other tissue to reach the tumor(s). Treatment with SBRT is typically complete in 5 or fewer sessions, called fractions.

MRI-Linac

The MRI-Linac is a recent development in radiation therapy. This device combines magnetic resonance imaging (MRI) with a radiation machine called a linear accelerator (LINAC). It is used in very specific circumstances, such as when giving SBRT. If the cancer spreads to an area where the tumor moves as a result of breathing, the MRI-Linac may be helpful. It can "track" and target the tumor in real time while you hold your breath at regular intervals during the treatment.

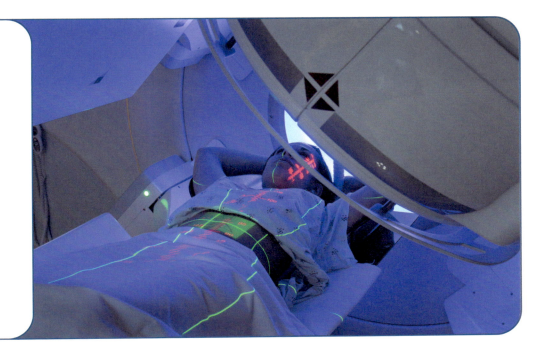

SBRT

SBRT is a specialized technique that delivers very high doses of radiation to one small location. It is usually used to treat rectal cancer that has spread to organs far from the rectum.

Stage 4 cancer in the liver or lungs

Resectable pMMR/MSS cancer

At this time, the preferred **first** treatment for resectable stage 4 cancers is chemotherapy with FOLFOX or CAPEOX. After chemotherapy, most people need more treatment that includes radiation therapy. Either short-course radiation therapy or chemoradiation is recommended.

After chemotherapy and any radiation therapy, the rectal tumor is resected and the liver or lung tumors are resected or destroyed using local therapies. This may be done at the same time, or as separate procedures. Sometimes chemotherapy works so well that radiation and surgery aren't needed. In this case, surveillance will begin.

A second option is to have either short-course radiation therapy or chemoradiation first, followed by chemotherapy. The extent of the cancer will be re-checked with imaging tests. Surgery is recommended next in most cases.

Unresectable pMMR/MSS cancer

If all areas of cancer cannot be safely removed using surgery or other local therapies, the cancer is **unresectable**. Treatment with chemotherapy is recommended. Recommended first-line regimens include:

> FOLFIRI

> FOLFOX

> CAPEOX

> FOLFIRINOX

Cancers that don't have *KRAS*, *NRAS*, or *BRAF* mutations are eligible for cetuximab or panitumumab in addition to chemotherapy. These are anti-EGFR therapies. For cancers with one of these mutations, bevacizumab (Avastin) may be added to chemotherapy.

While uncommon, systemic therapy may shrink the tumors enough to be removed or destroyed using surgery and local therapies. In this case, your doctor may suggest treatment that includes radiation therapy before proceeding with surgery. Short-course radiation therapy is preferred, but chemoradiation is also a recommended option. While uncommon, chemotherapy and radiation may work well enough that surgery isn't needed.

If the tumors do not become resectable during chemotherapy, systemic therapy is typically continued. The goal is to slow the growth and spread of the cancer. If there are a limited number of liver or lung tumors, treatment with local therapies may also be an option. If the rectal tumor grows during initial systemic therapy, you may first have chemoradiation or a short course of radiation to the rectal tumor before continuing systemic therapy.

If the cancer progresses, the regimen you receive next may be different from what you had before. One important factor is whether next-generation sequencing found any biomarkers. Regimens targeting specific biomarkers are listed in **Guide 4**.

If the cancer progresses through all available regimens, your options may include:

➤ Targeted therapy with fruquintinib (Fruzaqla)

➤ Chemotherapy with trifluridine and tipiracil (Lonsurf) (bevacizumab may be added)

➤ Targeted therapy with regorafenib (Stivarga)

All are tablets taken by mouth.

"

Be your own best advocate!"

Guide 4 Biomarker-based treatments for pMMR/MSS cancers	
BRAF **V600E mutation**	Encorafenib + (cetuximab or panitumumab)
HER2 amplification	• Trastuzumab (Herceptin) + pertuzumab, lapatinib, or tucatinib • Fam-trastuzumab deruxtecan-nxki (Enhertu)
KRAS **G12C mutation**	• Sotorasib (Lumakras) + cetuximab or panitumumab • Adagrasib (Krazati) + cetuximab or panitumumab
NTRK **gene fusion**	• Entrectinib (Rozlytrek) • Larotrectinib (Vitrakvi)
RET **gene fusion**	Selpercatinib (Retevmo)

dMMR/MSI-H or POLE/POLD1-mutated cancer

Treatment for **resectable** stage 4 rectal cancers with this biomarker starts with checkpoint inhibitor immunotherapy.

Immunotherapy is a type of systemic therapy. It increases the activity of parts of your immune system. This helps your body find and destroy cancer cells. If you are not eligible for a checkpoint inhibitor, having oxaliplatin-based chemotherapy is an option.

Assuming you haven't had treatment with a checkpoint inhibitor, currently recommended options include:

> Nivolumab (Opdivo), which may be given with ipilimumab (Yervoy)

> Pembrolizumab (Keytruda)

> Dostarlimab-gxly (Jemperli)

After immunotherapy, the extent of the cancer is re-checked with imaging tests. Most people need more treatment that includes radiation therapy. Short-course radiation therapy is preferred, but chemoradiation is also a recommended option.

After immunotherapy and any radiation therapy, the rectal tumor and the liver or lung tumors are removed using resection (surgery), often with other local therapies. The surgeries may be done at the same time, or as separate procedures.

Sometimes immunotherapy works so well that radiation and surgery aren't needed. In this case, surveillance will begin.

Immunotherapy side effects

Immune checkpoint inhibitors have unique side effects. Unlike other cancer treatments, the side effects of immunotherapy occur because the immune system is attacking healthy cells in the body. Learning to recognize possible side effects can help you notice reactions early and report them to your care team.

More information on the side effects of immune checkpoint inhibitors is available at NCCN.org/patientguidelines and on the NCCN Patient Guides for Cancer app.

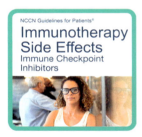

Checkpoint inhibitor immunotherapy is also recommended for **unresectable** stage 4 rectal cancers with this biomarker. Your doctor will check the extent of the cancer every 2 to 3 months. Surgery may become possible. Or you may continue immunotherapy or switch to a different systemic therapy.

Stage 4 cancer in the abdomen

Some people with metastatic rectal cancer will also form tumors in the thin layer of tissue that lines the abdomen, called the peritoneum. The peritoneum covers most of the organs in the abdomen.

Most people receive treatment with systemic therapy. The goal is to relieve or prevent symptoms. Your care team will select a regimen based on whether the tumor has any biomarkers and your overall health.

If the tumor is blocking stool from moving and leaving the body, the bowel needs to be unblocked before starting systemic therapy. This is done using a surgical technique or with a mesh metal tube called a stent.

Surveillance

If you have a complete response to treatment, surveillance for stage 4 rectal cancer includes:

> Colonoscopies
> Physical exams
> Carcinoembryonic antigen (CEA) blood tests
> Computed tomography (CT) scans

The recommended schedule is shown in **Guide 5.**

In addition to surveillance testing, a range of other care is important for cancer survivors. For more information, see the *Survivorship* chapter of this guide.

Guide 5 Surveillance after treatment for stage 4 rectal cancer	
Physical exam and CEA blood test	**First 2 years:** Every 3 to 6 months **Next 3 years:** Every 6 months
CT of chest, abdomen, and pelvis	**First 2 years:** Every 3 to 6 months **Next 3 years:** Every 6 to 12 months
Colonoscopy	If a total colonoscopy **wasn't** performed at diagnosis, it is recommended 3 to 6 months after surgery. If a total colonoscopy **was** performed at diagnosis, another is recommended 1 year after surgery. If no advanced cancerous polyps are found, your next will be in 3 years, and every 5 years after that.

Distant recurrence

After treatment for non-metastatic rectal cancer, the cancer may return and spread to the liver, lungs, or other areas. This is called a distant recurrence. Treatment with surgery and/or local therapies is recommended if all of the tumors can be totally removed. But, this is rare, and most people receive treatment with systemic therapy.

While uncommon, systemic therapy may shrink the tumors enough to be removed with surgery. If the cancer doesn't become resectable, systemic therapy is typically continued. The goal is to slow the growth and spread of the cancer.

Treatment recommendations are provided next according to the mismatch repair status of the cancer and whether resection is possible.

Unresectable pMMR/MSS cancer

If you've had recent treatment with FOLFOX or CAPEOX, you should not have more chemotherapy that includes oxaliplatin. Oxaliplatin can cause serious nerve damage. Your options for systemic therapy will depend, in part, on whether the cancer has any of the biomarkers listed below. Therapies are available that target these biomarkers.

> *HER2* amplification

> *KRAS* G12C mutation

> *BRAF* mutations

> *NTRK* gene fusion

> *RET* gene fusion

For cancers without biomarkers, chemotherapy with FOLFIRI or irinotecan is a recommended first-line option. Cancers that don't have *KRAS, NRAS,* or *BRAF* mutations are eligible for cetuximab (Erbitux) or panitumumab (Vectibix) in addition to chemotherapy. These are anti-EGFR therapies.

For cancers with *KRAS, NRAS,* or *BRAF* mutations, bevacizumab (Avastin), ziv-aflibercept (Zaltrap), or ramucirumab (Cyramza) may be added to chemotherapy.

Resectable pMMR/MSS cancer

If you've already had chemotherapy, one recommended option is resection (and/or treatment with local therapies) first, followed by either chemotherapy or observation. Observation is preferred for those who have already had treatment with oxaliplatin.

A second option is 2 to 3 months of chemotherapy first, followed by resection (and/or treatment with local therapies). More chemotherapy may follow.

If you haven't had any chemotherapy, resection (and/or treatment with local therapies) is often performed first, followed by chemotherapy with FOLFOX or CAPEOX. Capecitabine and 5-FU/leucovorin are options if needed.

A second option for those who haven't had any chemotherapy is 2 to 3 months of chemotherapy first, followed by resection and/or treatment with local therapies. More chemotherapy may follow.

Unresectable dMMR/MSI-H or POLE/POLD1-mutated cancer

If you are a candidate and haven't had immunotherapy, treatment with a checkpoint inhibitor is recommended. At this time, recommended options include:

> Nivolumab (Opdivo) with or without ipilimumab (Yervoy)

> Pembrolizumab (Keytruda)

> Dostarlimab-gxly (Jemperli)

Your doctor will check the extent of the cancer every 2 to 3 months. Surgery may become possible. Or, you may continue immunotherapy or switch to a different systemic therapy.

If you've already had immunotherapy, chemotherapy is typically given. A biologic may be included in the regimen. Or, if the cancer has any other biomarkers, targeted therapy may be an option.

Resectable dMMR/MSI-H or POLE/POLD1-mutated cancer

If you haven't had any immunotherapy, recommended options include:

> Immunotherapy, followed by observation or resection

> Resection followed by chemotherapy

Local therapies may be used together with resection, or used alone for very small tumors.

At this time, recommended checkpoint inhibitors for treating distant recurrence include:

> Nivolumab (Opdivo) with or without ipilimumab (Yervoy)

> Pembrolizumab (Keytruda)

> Dostarlimab-gxly (Jemperli)

If you've had prior immunotherapy, one recommended option is resection first, followed by either chemotherapy or observation. Observation is recommended for those who have already had treatment with oxaliplatin.

A second option is 2 to 3 months of chemotherapy first, followed by resection. More chemotherapy may follow.

Clinical trials

A clinical trial is a type of medical research study. After being developed and tested in a laboratory, potential new ways of fighting cancer need to be studied in people. If found to be safe and effective in a clinical trial, a drug, device, or treatment approach may be approved by the U.S. Food and Drug Administration (FDA).

Everyone with cancer should carefully consider all of the treatment options available for their cancer type, including standard treatments and clinical trials. Talk to your doctor about whether a clinical trial may make sense for you.

Phases

Most cancer clinical trials focus on treatment. Treatment trials are done in phases.

> **Phase 1** trials study the safety and side effects of an investigational drug or treatment approach.

> **Phase 2** trials study how well the drug or approach works against a specific type of cancer.

> **Phase 3** trials test the drug or approach against a standard treatment. If the results are good, it may be approved by the FDA.

> **Phase 4** trials study the long-term safety and benefit of an FDA-approved treatment.

Who can enroll?

Every clinical trial has rules for joining, called eligibility criteria. The rules may be about age, cancer type and stage, treatment history, or general health. These requirements ensure that participants are alike in specific ways

Finding a clinical trial

In the United States

NCCN Cancer Centers
NCCN.org/cancercenters

The National Cancer Institute (NCI)
cancer.gov/about-cancer/treatment/
clinical-trials/search

Worldwide

The U.S. National Library of Medicine (NLM)
clinicaltrials.gov

Need help finding a clinical trial?

NCI's Cancer Information Service (CIS)
1.800.4.CANCER (1.800.422.6237)
cancer.gov/contact

and that the trial is as safe as possible for the participants.

Informed consent

Clinical trials are managed by a group of experts called a research team. The research team will review the study with you in detail, including its purpose and the risks and benefits of joining. All of this information is also provided in an informed consent form. Read the form carefully and ask questions before signing it. Take time to discuss with family, friends, or others you trust. Keep in mind that you can leave and seek treatment outside of the clinical trial at any time.

Start the conversation

Don't wait for your doctor to bring up clinical trials. Start the conversation and learn about all of your treatment options. If you find a study that you may be eligible for, ask your treatment team if you meet the requirements. Try not to be discouraged if you cannot join. New clinical trials are always becoming available.

Frequently asked questions

There are many myths and misconceptions surrounding clinical trials. The possible benefits and risks are not well understood by many with cancer.

Will I get a placebo?
Placebos (inactive versions of real medicines) are almost never used alone in cancer clinical trials. It is common to receive either a placebo with a standard treatment, or a new drug with a standard treatment. You will be informed, verbally and in writing, if a placebo is part of a clinical trial before you enroll.

Are clinical trials free?
There is no fee to enroll in a clinical trial. The study sponsor pays for research-related costs, including the study drug. You may, however, have costs indirectly related to the trial, such as the cost of transportation or child care due to extra appointments. During the trial, you will continue to receive standard cancer care. This care is billed to—and often covered by—insurance. You are responsible for copays and any costs for this care that are not covered by your insurance.

Key points

> Everyone with metastatic rectal cancer should have biomarker tumor testing for *RAS* mutations, *BRAF* mutations, *HER2* amplification, and mismatch repair deficiency (if not already performed).

> Next-generation sequencing (NGS) can find other, rare biomarkers for which targeted treatments may be available.

> Treatment options for metastatic rectal cancer may include local therapies, such as thermal ablation and SBRT.

> Stage 4 cancer that cannot be removed with surgery and/or local therapies is treated with systemic therapy.

> For those who are eligible, checkpoint inhibitor immunotherapy is recommended for mismatch repair deficient (dMMR) and *POLE/POLD1*-mutated metastatic cancers.

> Supportive care is available for everyone with cancer to help with symptoms and make you more comfortable.

> Clinical trials provide access to investigational treatments that may, in time, be approved by the FDA.

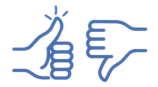

Let us know what you think!

Please take a moment to complete an online survey about the
NCCN Guidelines for Patients.

NCCN.org/patients/response

5
Survivorship

Survivorship focuses on the physical, emotional, and financial issues faced by cancer survivors. Managing the long-term side effects of cancer and its treatment and living a healthy lifestyle are important parts of survivorship.

Your primary care provider

After finishing cancer treatment, your oncologist and primary care provider should work together to make sure you get needed follow-up care. Ask your oncologist for a written survivorship care plan. Ideally, the plan will include:

> A summary of your cancer treatment history

> A description of possible late- and long-term side effects

> Recommendations for monitoring for the return of cancer

> Clear roles and responsibilities for your providers

> Recommendations on your overall health and well-being

Caregivers need to take care of themselves first. It's not selfish. It's necessary to get through the tough months or years that lie ahead."

Help with side effects

Rectal cancer survivors may experience both short- and long-term health effects of cancer and its treatment. The effects depend in part on the treatment(s) received. Surgery, anti-cancer medicines, and radiation therapy all have unique potential side effects.

Bowel changes

Surgery that involves removing all or part of the rectum is called a low anterior resection (LAR). This type of surgery often causes changes to bowel function, such as:

> Overall increase in bowel movements

> Urgent need to pass stool

> Having many (possibly watery) bowel movements over the course of a few hours (stool clustering)

> Irregular and unpredictable bowel movements

> Inability to control bowel movements (fecal incontinence)

> Increase in gas (flatulence)

Together these symptoms are referred to as low anterior resection syndrome (LARS).

Loperamide (Imodium) is an over-the-counter anti-diarrheal medicine. It can help with stool clustering and incontinence. Exercises that strengthen the muscles in the pelvic floor can help with urgency and stool incontinence.

Changes to diet can also help with LARS symptoms. Eat foods high in insoluble (not soluble) fiber and use fiber supplements. Psyllium-based products (like Metamucil) may help slow and thicken the stool. Ask your treatment team for a list of foods that may help or worsen bowel changes after low anterior resection. Many people find that protective undergarments provide peace of mind.

Nerve damage

The chemotherapy drug oxaliplatin can damage nerves in your fingers and toes. Symptoms include numbness, cramping, tingling, or pain in these areas. Acupuncture and heat may help. If you have painful nerve damage, a drug called duloxetine (Cymbalta) may help. If the pain is persistent, talk to your doctor about seeing a pain management specialist.

Ostomy care

If you have an ostomy, you may want to join an ostomy support group. Another option is to see a health care provider that specializes in ostomy care, such as an ostomy nurse.

People with ostomies can still live very active lifestyles. However, it's a good idea to talk to an ostomy professional before doing any intense physical activity.

Sexual health

Many people experience sexual side effects after chemotherapy and radiation. For those with a penis, this could mean difficulty getting an erection. Those with a vagina may experience vaginal dryness and pain during sex.

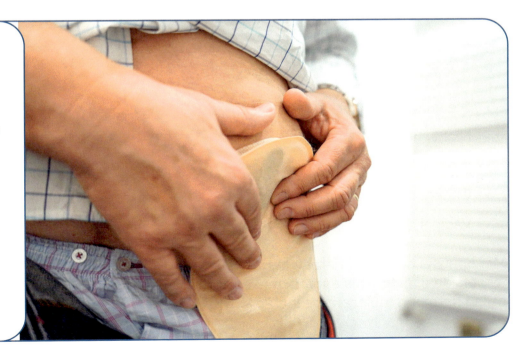

Ostomy care

You can still live an active lifestyle with an ostomy. Joining a support group or seeing an ostomy nurse can help you learn more about living with an ostomy.

Radiation therapy to the pelvis can cause the vagina to become shorter and more narrow. This is called vaginal stenosis. Vaginal stenosis can make it uncomfortable or even painful to have sex, or to have vaginal examinations by a doctor. Vaginal dilator therapy can help. A vaginal dilator is a device used to gradually stretch or widen the vagina. Vaginal dilators are not one-size-fits-all. Different sizes are available, as are kits containing different size devices. The size of the dilator can be increased over time as the vagina lengthens and widens. Use of a vaginal dilator can begin as soon as you are healed after treatment.

Menopausal hormone therapy

The ovaries make hormones needed for menstruation and natural pregnancy. Radiation damages the ovaries, causing hormone levels to drop. This is known as premature ovarian insufficiency (POI) or radiation-induced premature menopause. It causes infertility and may also cause symptoms of menopause, including:

- > Stopping of periods
- > Hot flashes
- > Sleeping problems
- > Night sweats
- > Weight gain
- > Changes in mood
- > Vaginal dryness

Menopausal hormone therapy may help lessen these side effects. This approach used to be called hormone replacement therapy or HRT.

One option is systemic combination therapy. Both estrogen and progestogen are given, usually either as a pill or a patch placed on the skin. The hormones travel throughout the body in the bloodstream. Progestogen is included because giving estrogen by itself can increase the risk of uterine cancer in those with a uterus.

Another option for menopausal hormone therapy is vaginal estrogen cream or tablets. This type may be the best option for symptoms that mainly affect the vagina, such as dryness.

Discussion with a specialized menopausal symptom team may be helpful to determine whether this treatment is right for you.

Paying for care

Cancer survivors face a unique financial burden. Paying for doctor visits, tests, and treatments can become unmanageable, especially for those with little or no health insurance. You may also have costs not directly related to treatment, such as travel expenses and the cost of childcare or missed work.

The term financial toxicity is used to describe the problems patients face related to the cost of medical care. Financial toxicity can affect your quality of life and access to needed health care. If you need help paying for your cancer care, financial assistance may be available. Talk with a patient navigator, your treatment team's social worker, and your hospital's financial services department.

Healthy habits

It is important to keep up with other aspects of your health after cancer treatment. Steps you can take to help prevent other health problems and to improve your quality of life are described next.

Cancer screening

Get screened for other types of cancer, such as breast, prostate, and skin cancer. Your primary care doctor can tell you what cancer screening tests you should have based on your age and risk level.

Other health care

Get other recommended health care for your age, such as blood pressure screening, hepatitis C screening, and immunizations (like the flu shot).

Diet and exercise

Try to exercise for at least 150 minutes per week. Alcohol may increase the risk of certain cancers. Drink little to no alcohol. A low glycemic load (GL) diet may help prevent the return of rectal cancer. Low GL foods cause a slower and smaller rise in blood sugar levels compared to other carbohydrate-containing foods. Talk to your doctor about a low glycemic load diet.

Aspirin

Talk to your doctor about the possible risks and benefits of long-term aspirin therapy to help prevent the return of colorectal cancers.

Quit smoking

If you smoke or vape, quit! Tell your care team. They can help.

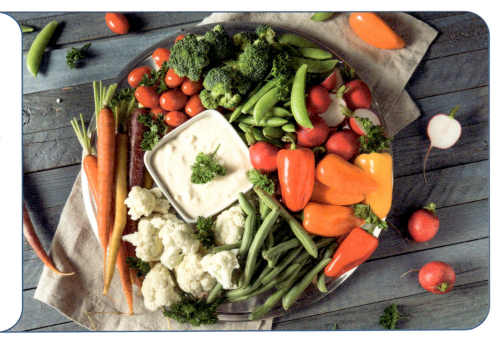

Experts recommend eating a healthy diet, especially one that includes a lot of plant-based foods (vegetables, fruits, and whole grains).

More information

For more information on cancer survivorship, the following are available at NCCN.org/patientguidelines:

> *Survivorship Care for Healthy Living*
> *Survivorship Care for Cancer-Related Late and Long-Term Effects*

These resources address topics relevant to cancer survivors, including:

> Anxiety, depression, and distress
> Fatigue
> Pain
> Sexual health
> Sleep problems
> Healthy lifestyles
> Immunizations
> Employment, insurance, and disability concerns

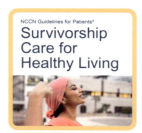
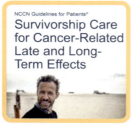

"

Self advocate and ask questions. Your medical team's goal is to save your life. Become informed and also be a partner in your care. Speak up. Now is not the time to be shy. If you don't understand something or want to know if other options are available, ask questions. Don't leave an appointment if you have something you want to say or ask. Don't feel like you should know the answers."

6
Making treatment decisions

It's important to be comfortable with the cancer treatment you choose. This choice starts with having an open and honest conversation with your doctor.

It's your choice

In shared decision-making, you and your care team share information, discuss the options, and agree on a treatment plan. It starts with an open and honest conversation between you and your care team.

Treatment decisions are very personal. What is important to you may not be important to someone else. Some things that may play a role in your decision-making:

> What you want and how that might differ from what others want

> Your religious and spiritual beliefs

> Your feelings about certain treatments

> Your feelings about pain or side effects

> Cost of treatment, travel to treatment centers, and time away from school or work

> Quality of life and length of life

> How active you are and the activities that are important to you

Think about what you want from treatment. Discuss openly the risks and benefits of specific treatments and procedures. Weigh options

and share concerns with your care team. If you take the time to build a relationship with your care team, it will help you feel supported when considering options and making treatment decisions.

Second opinion

It is normal to want to start treatment as soon as possible. While cancer can't be ignored, there is time to have another doctor review your test results and suggest a treatment plan. This is called getting a second opinion, and it's a normal part of cancer care. Even doctors get second opinions!

Things you can do to prepare:

> Check with your insurance company about its rules on second opinions. There may be out-of-pocket costs to see doctors who are not part of your insurance plan.

> Make plans to have copies of all your records sent to the doctor you will see for your second opinion.

Support groups

Many people diagnosed with cancer find support groups to be helpful. Support groups often include people at different stages of treatment. Some people may be newly diagnosed, while others may be finished with treatment. If your hospital or community doesn't have support groups for people with cancer, check out the websites listed in this book.

Questions to ask

Possible questions to ask your care team are listed on the following pages. Feel free to use these questions or come up with your own.

Questions about treatment

1. Do you consult NCCN recommendations when considering options?

2. Are you suggesting options other than what NCCN recommends? If yes, why?

3. Do your suggested options include clinical trials? Please explain why.

4. How do my age, health, and other factors affect my options?

5. What if I am pregnant, or planning to become pregnant in the future?

6. What are the benefits and risks of each option? Does any option offer a cure or long-term cancer control?

7. How much will treatment cost? What does my insurance cover?

8. How long do I have to decide about treatment?

9. Who can I call outside of office hours if I have an urgent problem with my cancer or my cancer treatment?

10. When will I know the results from my genetic testing or biomarker testing?

Questions about non-metastatic rectal cancer

1. Do I need surgery? If so, what type?

2. Is the cancer locally advanced? If so, will I have total neoadjuvant therapy?

3. How likely is it that surgery will be possible after total neoadjuvant therapy?

4. Which side effects of surgery are most likely?

5. How do I prepare for surgery? Do I have to stop taking any of my medicines? Are there foods I will have to avoid?

6. When will I be able to return to my normal activities?

7. Is home care after treatment needed? If yes, what type?

8. What follow-up testing is needed for my cancer stage?

9. How likely is the cancer to return after treatment? Can I do anything to lower the risk?

10. If the cancer does return, what is the recommended treatment?

Questions about stage 4 rectal cancer

1. Where has the cancer spread?

2. Am I a candidate for surgery? If not, is it possible that I'll become a candidate?

3. What treatment will I have before, during, or after surgery?

4. Am I a candidate for treatment with local therapies? Did an interventional oncologist/radiologist review my case?

5. Which systemic therapy regimen do you recommend for me? Why?

6. How will you know if systemic therapy is working? What if it stops working?

7. Does my cancer have any biomarkers? How does this affect my options?

8. What is my prognosis?

9. What can be done to prevent or relieve the side effects of treatment?

10. Am I a candidate for a clinical trial? Do you know of one I can join?

Questions about resources and support

1. Who can I talk to about help with housing, food, and other basic needs?

2. What help is available for transportation, childcare, and home care?

3. How much will I have to pay for treatment?

4. What help is available to pay for medicines and treatment?

5. What other services are available to me and my caregivers?

6. How can I connect with others and build a support system?

7. How can I find in-person or online support?

8. Who can help me with my concerns about missing work or school?

9. Who can I talk to if I don't feel safe at home, at work, or in my neighborhood?

10. How can I get help to stop smoking or vaping?

Resources

Bone Marrow & Cancer Foundation
Bonemarrow.org

Cancer*Care*
Cancercare.org

Cancer Hope Network
Cancerhopenetwork.org

Colorectal Cancer Alliance
ccalliance.org

Fight Colorectal Cancer
fightcolorectalcancer.org

HPV Cancers Alliance
Hpvca.org

Love Your Buns
Loveyourbuns.org

National Coalition for Cancer Survivorship
canceradvocacy.org

Paltown
Paltown.org

Triage Cancer
Triagecancer.org

U.S. National Library of Medicine Clinical Trials Database
clinicaltrials.gov

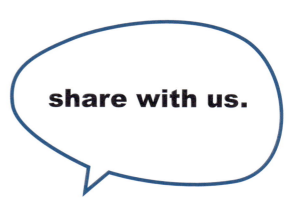

Take our survey and help make the NCCN Guidelines for Patients better for everyone!

NCCN.org/patients/comments

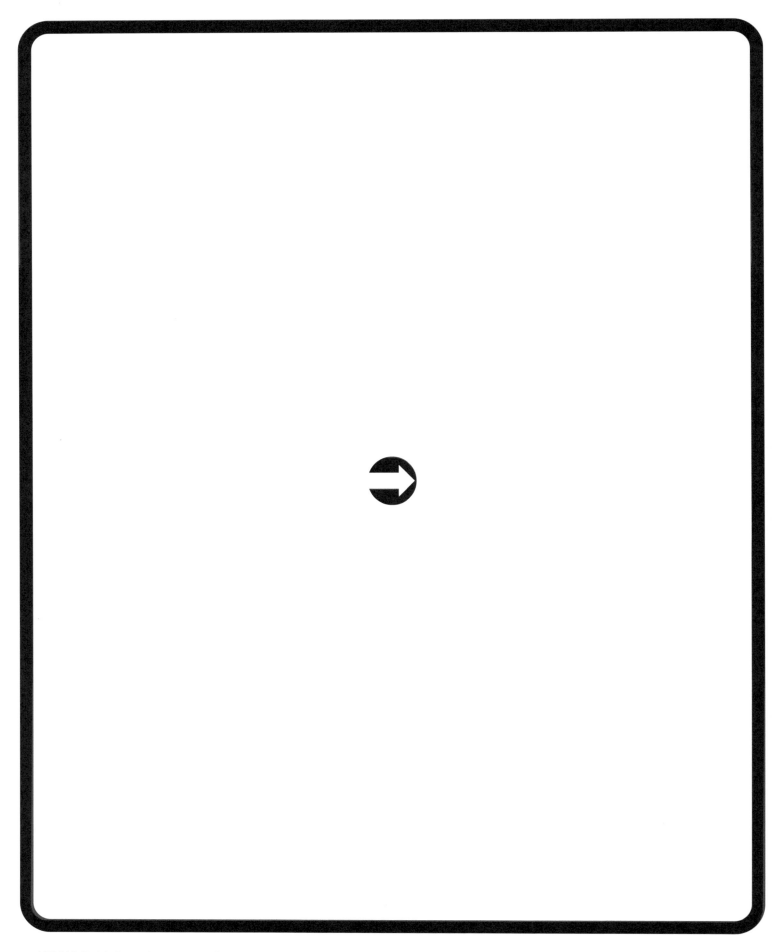

Words to know

ablation
A type of local therapy used to destroy tumors in the liver or lungs. Also called image-guided thermal ablation.

adenocarcinoma
Cancer in cells that line organs and make fluids or hormones. The most common type of rectal cancer.

adenoma
The most common type of colorectal polyp and the most likely to form cancer cells. Also called adenomatous polyp.

biomarkers
Specific features of cancer cells used to guide treatment. Biomarkers are often mutations (changes) in the DNA of the cancer cells.

CAPEOX
A chemotherapy regimen that includes capecitabine and oxaliplatin.

carcinoembryonic antigen (CEA)
A protein that gets released by some tumors and can be detected in blood.

colon
The first and longest section of the large bowel. Unused food is turned into stool in the colon.

colostomy
Surgery to connect a part of the colon to the outside of the abdomen and that allows stool to drain into a bag.

embolization
Blockage of blood flow to a tumor with beads that emit either chemotherapy or radiation.

endoscopic submucosal dissection (ESD)
A minimally invasive type of surgery used to remove small rectal tumors in one piece. Also called endoscopic mucosal resection (EMR).

external beam radiation therapy (EBRT)
Treatment with high-energy rays received from a machine outside the body.

familial adenomatous polyposis (FAP)
An inherited medical condition that increases the risk of rectal cancer.

FOLFIRI
A chemotherapy regimen used for some advanced colorectal cancers. Includes leucovorin calcium, fluorouracil, and irinotecan.

FOLFIRINOX
A chemotherapy regimen used for some advanced colorectal cancers. Includes leucovorin calcium (folinic acid), fluorouracil, irinotecan, and oxaliplatin.

FOLFOX
A chemotherapy regimen that includes leucovorin calcium, fluorouracil, and oxaliplatin.

interventional oncology/radiology
A medical specialty that uses imaging techniques to deliver minimally invasive cancer treatments.

large intestine (bowel)
A long tube-shaped organ that forms the last part of the digestive system. Includes the colon, rectum, and anus.

lymph
A clear fluid containing white blood cells.

lymph node
Small groups of special disease-fighting cells located throughout the body.

metastasis
The spread of cancer cells from the first (primary) tumor to a distant site.

mismatch repair deficiency (dMMR)/high microsatellite instability (MSI-H)
A biomarker (feature) of some colorectal cancers that is used to guide treatment. All colorectal cancers should be tested for this biomarker.

mismatch repair proficient (pMMR)/ microsatellite stable (MSS)
Describes cancers that don't have the mismatch repair deficiency (dMMR) biomarker.

pathologist
A doctor who specializes in testing cells and tissue to find disease.

polyp
An overgrowth of cells on the inner lining of the colon wall. Pedunculated polyps are shaped like mushrooms with a stalk. Sessile polyps are flat.

portal vein embolization
The blood vessel to the liver tumor is blocked causing the healthy part of the liver to grow larger.

rectum
An organ in the digestive system that holds stool until it exits the body through the anus.

recurrence
The return of cancer after a cancer-free period.

resectable
Describes a cancer that can be safely removed using surgery.

stereotactic body radiation therapy (SBRT)
A highly specialized type of radiation therapy. May be used to treat rectal cancer that has spread to the liver, lungs, or bone.

supportive care
Treatment for the symptoms or health conditions caused by cancer or cancer treatment.

surgical margin
The normal tissue around the edge of a tumor removed during surgery.

systemic therapy
The use of medicines that enter the bloodstream. Chemotherapy, targeted therapy, and immunotherapy are examples.

unresectable
Describes a cancer that cannot be safely removed using surgery.

NCCN Contributors

This patient guide is based on the NCCN Clinical Practice Guidelines in Oncology (NCCN Guidelines®) for Rectal cancer, Version 1.2024. It was adapted, reviewed, and published with help from the following people:

Dorothy A. Shead, MS
Senior Director
Patient Information Operations

Erin Vidic, MA
Senior Medical Writer, Patient Information

Laura Phillips
Graphic Artist

The NCCN Clinical Practice Guidelines in Oncology (NCCN Guidelines®) for Rectal cancer, Version 1.2024 were developed by the following NCCN Panel Members:

Al B. Benson, III, MD/Chair
Robert H. Lurie Comprehensive Cancer Center of Northwestern University

Alan P. Venook, MD/Vice-Chair
UCSF Helen Diller Family Comprehensive Cancer Center

Mohamed Adam, MD
UCSF Helen Diller Family Comprehensive Cancer Center

Yi-Jen Chen, MD, PhD
City of Hope National Medical Center

Kristen K. Ciombor, MD
Vanderbilt-Ingram Cancer Center

Stacey Cohen, MD
Fred Hutchinson Cancer Center

Harry S. Cooper, MD
Fox Chase Cancer Center

Dustin Deming, MD
University of Wisconsin Carbone Cancer Center

Ignacio Garrido-Laguna, MD, PhD
Huntsman Cancer Institute at the University of Utah

Jean L. Grem, MD
Fred & Pamela Buffett Cancer Center

Paul Haste, MD
Indiana University Melvin and Bren Simon Comprehensive Cancer Center

J. Randolph Hecht, MD
UCLA Jonsson Comprehensive Cancer Center

Sarah Hoffe, MD
Moffitt Cancer Center

Steven Hunt, MD
Siteman Cancer Center at Barnes-Jewish Hospital and Washington University School of Medicine

*Hisham Hussan, MD
UC Davis Comprehensive Cancer Center

*Kimberly L. Johung, MD, PhD
Yale Cancer Center/Smilow Cancer Hospital

Nora Joseph, MD
University of Michigan Rogel Cancer Center

Natalie Kirilcuk, MD
Stanford Cancer Institute

Smitha Krishnamurthi, MD
Case Comprehensive Cancer Center/ University Hospitals Seidman Cancer Center and Cleveland Clinic Taussig Cancer Institute

Midhun Malla, MD, MS
O'Neal Comprehensive Cancer Center at UAB

Jennifer K. Maratt, MD
Indiana University Melvin and Bren Simon Comprehensive Cancer Center

Wells A. Messersmith, MD
University of Colorado Cancer Center

Jeffrey Meyerhardt, MD, MPH
Dana-Farber Brigham and Women's Cancer Center

Eric D. Miller, MD, PhD
The Ohio State University Comprehensive Cancer Center - James Cancer Hospital and Solove Research Institute

Mary F. Mulcahy, MD
Robert H. Lurie Comprehensive Cancer Center of Northwestern University

*Steven Nurkin, MD, MS
Roswell Park Comprehensive Cancer Center

Michael J. Overman, MD
The University of Texas MD Anderson Cancer Center

Aparna Parikh, MD, MS
Mass General Cancer Center

Hitendra Patel, MD
UC San Diego Moores Cancer Center

Katrina Pedersen, MD, MS
Siteman Cancer Center at Barnes-Jewish Hospital and Washington University School of Medicine

Leonard Saltz, MD
Memorial Sloan Kettering Cancer Center

*Charles Schneider, MD
Abramson Cancer Center at the University of Pennsylvania

David Shibata, MD
The University of Tennessee Health Science Center

Benjamin Shogan, MD
The UChicago Medicine Comprehensive Cancer Center

John M. Skibber, MD
The University of Texas MD Anderson Cancer Center

Constantinos T. Sofocleous, MD, PhD
Memorial Sloan Kettering Cancer Center

Anna Tavakkoli, MD, MSc
UT Southwestern Simmons Comprehensive Cancer Center

Christopher G. Willett, MD
Duke Cancer Institute

*Christina Wu, MD
Mayo Clinic Comprehensive Cancer Center

NCCN

Frankie Jones
Guidelines Layout Specialist

Lisa Gurski, PhD
Manager, Licensed Clinical Content

Jenna Snedeker, MS, ASCP
Associate Scientist/Medical Writer

* Reviewed this patient guide. For disclosures, visit NCCN.org/disclosures.

NCCN Cancer Centers

Abramson Cancer Center
at the University of Pennsylvania
Philadelphia, Pennsylvania
800.789.7366 • pennmedicine.org/cancer

Case Comprehensive Cancer Center/
University Hospitals Seidman Cancer Center and
Cleveland Clinic Taussig Cancer Institute
Cleveland, Ohio
UH Seidman Cancer Center
800.641.2422 • uhhospitals.org/services/cancer-services
CC Taussig Cancer Institute
866.223.8100 • my.clevelandclinic.org/departments/cancer
Case CCC
216.844.8797 • case.edu/cancer

City of Hope National Medical Center
Duarte, California
800.826.4673 • cityofhope.org

Dana-Farber/Brigham and Women's Cancer Center |
Mass General Cancer Center
Boston, Massachusetts
877-442-3324 • youhaveus.org
617.726.5130 • massgeneral.org/cancer-center

Duke Cancer Institute
Durham, North Carolina
888.275.3853 • dukecancerinstitute.org

Fox Chase Cancer Center
Philadelphia, Pennsylvania
888.369.2427 • foxchase.org

Fred & Pamela Buffett Cancer Center
Omaha, Nebraska
402.559.5600 • unmc.edu/cancercenter

Fred Hutchinson Cancer Center
Seattle, Washington
206.667.5000 • fredhutch.org

Huntsman Cancer Institute at the University of Utah
Salt Lake City, Utah
800.824.2073 • healthcare.utah.edu/huntsmancancerinstitute

Indiana University Melvin and Bren Simon
Comprehensive Cancer Center
Indianapolis, Indiana
888.600.4822 • www.cancer.iu.edu

Mayo Clinic Comprehensive Cancer Center
Phoenix/Scottsdale, Arizona
Jacksonville, Florida
Rochester, Minnesota
480.301.8000 • Arizona
904.953.0853 • Florida
507.538.3270 • Minnesota
mayoclinic.org/cancercenter

Memorial Sloan Kettering Cancer Center
New York, New York
800.525.2225 • mskcc.org

Moffitt Cancer Center
Tampa, Florida
888.663.3488 • moffitt.org

O'Neal Comprehensive Cancer Center at UAB
Birmingham, Alabama
800.822.0933 • uab.edu/onealcancercenter

Robert H. Lurie Comprehensive Cancer
Center of Northwestern University
Chicago, Illinois
866.587.4322 • cancer.northwestern.edu

Roswell Park Comprehensive Cancer Center
Buffalo, New York
877.275.7724 • roswellpark.org

Siteman Cancer Center at Barnes-Jewish Hospital
and Washington University School of Medicine
St. Louis, Missouri
800.600.3606 • siteman.wustl.edu

St. Jude Children's Research Hospital/
The University of Tennessee Health Science Center
Memphis, Tennessee
866.278.5833 • stjude.org
901.448.5500 • uthsc.edu

Stanford Cancer Institute
Stanford, California
877.668.7535 • cancer.stanford.edu

The Ohio State University Comprehensive Cancer Center -
James Cancer Hospital and Solove Research Institute
Columbus, Ohio
800.293.5066 • cancer.osu.edu

The Sidney Kimmel Comprehensive
Cancer Center at Johns Hopkins
Baltimore, Maryland
410.955.8964
www.hopkinskimmelcancercenter.org

The UChicago Medicine Comprehensive Cancer Center
Chicago, Illinois
773.702.1000 • uchicagomedicine.org/cancer

The University of Texas MD Anderson Cancer Center
Houston, Texas
844.269.5922 • mdanderson.org

UC Davis Comprehensive Cancer Center
Sacramento, California
916.734.5959 • 800.770.9261
health.ucdavis.edu/cancer

UC San Diego Moores Cancer Center
La Jolla, California
858.822.6100 • cancer.ucsd.edu

UCLA Jonsson Comprehensive Cancer Center
Los Angeles, California
310.825.5268 • uclahealth.org/cancer

UCSF Helen Diller Family Comprehensive Cancer Center
San Francisco, California
800.689.8273 • cancer.ucsf.edu

University of Colorado Cancer Center
Aurora, Colorado
720.848.0300 • coloradocancercenter.org

University of Michigan Rogel Cancer Center
Ann Arbor, Michigan
800.865.1125 • rogelcancercenter.org

University of Wisconsin Carbone Cancer Center
Madison, Wisconsin
608.265.1700 • uwhealth.org/cancer

UT Southwestern Simmons Comprehensive Cancer Center
Dallas, Texas
214.648.3111 • utsouthwestern.edu/simmons

Vanderbilt-Ingram Cancer Center
Nashville, Tennessee
877.936.8422 • vicc.org

Yale Cancer Center/Smilow Cancer Hospital
New Haven, Connecticut
855.4.SMILOW • yalecancercenter.org

Index

Made in United States
Troutdale, OR
06/08/2025